Massage - The Feel Good Medicine Without All the Bad Side Effects

I0417299

The Complete Guide to Treating Numerous Medical Conditions Using Massage Therapy

RON KNESS

Contents

Disclaimer

This publication is for informational purposes only and is not intended as medical advice. Medical advice should always be obtained from a qualified medical professional for any health conditions or symptoms associated with them.

Every possible effort has been made in preparing and researching this material. We make no warranties with respect to the accuracy, applicability of its contents or any omissions.

See your healthcare professional before starting any diet, health or exercise program!

Introduction – What Is Massage Therapy?

Massage therapy is considered to be one of the oldest methods of healing, with the practice dating back to around 2000 B.C. Although there weren't so many different massage techniques back then as there are now, the idea behind it was essentially the same.

The practice of massage therapy refers to the application of 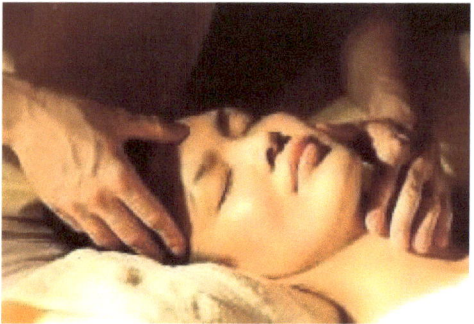 pressure to the soft tissues of your body using different techniques, such as friction, kneading and vibration. This pressure is applied to manipulate your soft body tissues (muscles, ligaments, tendons, connective tissue), thus improving one's health and well-being.

There are many reasons to seek massage therapy. Some of the most notable health benefits of massages include:

- Reduced anxiety and stress

- Pain relief

- Improved strength of the immune system

- Relaxation of muscles

- Enhanced mood

- Improved heart health

- Enhanced blood flow

- Lower blood pressure

- Reduced risk of depression

Many professional and amateur athletes get regular massages to improve athletic performance and help with injury recovery.

According to the American Massage Therapy Association (AMTA), massage is a therapy that promotes complete and total wellness and health of both the mind and body. According to an AMTA surveyed conducted in 2015, 88% of participants viewed massage as beneficial to overall health and wellness.

In modern times, massage is no longer a mere luxury, but the most widely used type of alternative medicine therapy in hospitals for mental health, pain management, stress reduction, and general wellness.

Popular Forms of Massage

Swedish Massage

Swedish massage is the most common type of massage therapy offered in the United States. If you haven't taken part in massage therapy before, then Swedish massage is the place to start. The main goal of this technique is to help relax your superficial muscles and improve blood circulation.

Swedish massage therapy is based around five different massage movements – kneading movements, vibration, sliding movements, percussion, and rubbing.

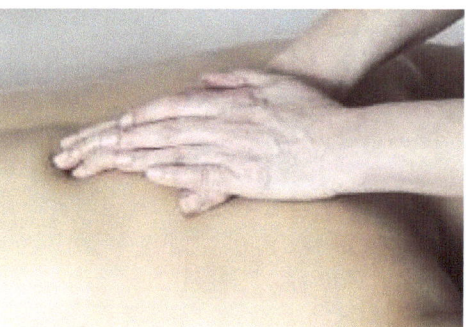

Traditionally, Swedish massage also includes both active and passive joint movements and stretching with the assistance of your massage therapist.

Considering that this type of massage will improve blood circulation, it will have a positive effect on your soft tissues. Namely, good circulation will stimulate your body to clean and nourish soft tissues, such as the skin and muscles. Swedish massage is also known to significantly reduce stress, help heal injuries and relieve pain.

Swedish massage is considered to be the foundation for many other types of massage therapies, including deep tissue, sports, and aromatherapy massage methods.

Although most people choose to take part in a 60-minute Swedish massage, it might be better to book a 90-minute session, as it will give your therapist more time to properly work on your muscle tissue.

Deep Tissue Massage

Although it's somewhat based on Swedish massage therapy, deep tissue massage is different because it was designed to reach the deeper layers of your muscles and the connective tissues around them.

If you have ever taken part in a Swedish massage therapy, then deep tissue massage might feel similar, mainly since the strokes are often the same or incredibly similar. The main difference is in the pressure being applied, where the therapist uses more pressure to apply deeper strokes to physically break down muscle adhesions that are the cause of your pain, inflammation, and limited range of motion. Muscle adhesions can also cause poor circulation.

A typical deep tissue massage session starts off with the therapist applying light pressure to properly warm up your muscles, followed by deeper and stronger pressure. A regular deep tissue massage session lasts from 45 to 60 minutes. This massage technique is usually used to treat various injuries and chronic muscle pain.

Shiatsu

Shiatsu is a massage technique that originated in Japan, but has become extremely popular in almost all parts of the world. When translated, shiatsu means "finger pressure," which is a great way to describe this technique.

A shiatsu massage session involves the therapist using fingers, thumbs, palms, elbows, hands, knees, and/or feet in order to apply pressure to certain parts of your body. The therapist will also focus on stretching and rotating your joints, limbs, and pressure points.

The way eastern medicine views healing is much different from how it's viewed in western medicine. While western medicine usually suggests that you take pills in order to fix your health problems, eastern medicine focuses on forming a balance between your mind and body in order to heal yourself.

This is why the theory behind shiatsu is much different from the previous two techniques that we've mentioned. Namely, shiatsu revolves around the belief that your body is completely made up of energy, and when that energy is blocked, you experience pain and discomfort. By participating in a shiatsu massage, you will remove these blockages and help the energy spread evenly throughout your body.

The theory behind shiatsu suggests that by balancing your energy, your body will heal itself, which will provide relief for both your mind and body.

Some of the most notable health benefits of shiatsu include pain relief, improved blood circulation, relaxation, and a decreased risk in developing arthritis. It also has a very positive impact on your mental health. Shiatsu will not only lower your stress levels, but it will also improve your mood.

Aromatherapy Massage

Aromatherapy is the use of essential oils that's scents stimulates the olfactory system, bringing various benefits including, stress relief, relaxation, and a variety of other health benefits.

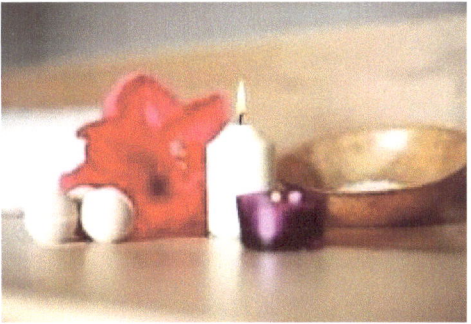

Aromatherapy is commonly used to help you unwind, cure minor ailments, reduce your stress levels, improve your mood, and renew your energy. There are a few ways to include aromatherapy into your life, such as inhaling essential oils, adding them to your bath, and mixing them with a carrier oil to be used in massage therapy.

Aromatherapy massage is the perfect option for you if you're not in the mood for a strenuous muscle-kneading massage. This massage technique doesn't really revolve around the therapist physically working out all the sore spots in your body. Instead, the goal of aromatherapy massage is simply to help relax your mind and body. This is, of course achieved with the use of essential oils, which are basically highly concentrated plant essences.

Although you will experience the benefits of essential oils through contact with your skin, inhaling and absorbing them through your mouth and nose is what will actually help you get the most benefits. It's not uncommon for different therapists to use different massage technique during aromatherapy massage.

Hot Stone Massage

Hot stone massage refers to a technique in which smooth, heated stones are positioned on specific parts of your body in order to maximize the healing effect of the massage.

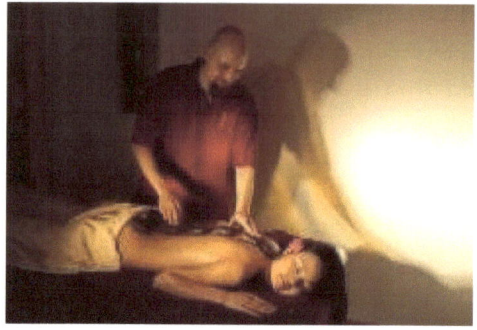

The therapist may also use these heated stones as an extension of their hands, meaning that they won't just leave the stones on your body, but that they will actually apply pressure with them.

This type of massage therapy is based on a technique Native Americans use to treat muscle aches. The purpose of these stone is to relax tense muscles, which is easily achieved through the weight and warmth of the stones. River rocks are mostly used because they are notably smooth.

If you're feeling muscle tension but would like to get a lighter massage, then you should definitely book a hot stone massage session. Most people find the warmth of the stones used in this massage to be very relaxing and comforting.

This technique is used to treat anxiety, insomnia, back pain, osteoarthritis, and depression. Despite what some people may think, this type of massage is not painful. If, however, you feel that the stones or your body is too hot, make sure to inform your therapist immediately.

Thai Massage

Thai massage is based on the same belief as shiatsu, which is that your body is completely made up of energy. By taking part in Thai massage, you will achieve a state of deep relaxation, which can improve your emotional state and can even help change your personal outlook on life in a positive way.

Thai massage is basically a mixture of assisted yoga postures, acupressure, and Ayurveda.

It is different from most other massages in the sense that it doesn't involve the use of lotion or oil. It is also not performed on an elevated massage table, like most massages. Instead, it is performed on a futon or padded mat on the floor.

Throughout the duration of the massage, you remain fully clothed. During a Thai massage session, you can expect the therapist to use their knees, legs, hands, and feet, to move you into different yoga-like poses in order to provide your body with the stretching it needs.

Thai massage offers you unbeatable stretching, which is just one of the benefits it provides. Other notable benefits include improved mood, decreased cortisol levels, improved circulation, pain relief, and stress relief.

Note that Thai massage is not your typical massage therapy. It can be invigorating and painful. However, as long as you co-operate with your therapist and always let them know how much pain you're experiencing (if you are experiencing any pain), then they will be able to adjust the movements and pressure accordingly.

Reflexology

Most people believe that reflexology is just a fancy term for foot massage. However, reflexology is something much more.

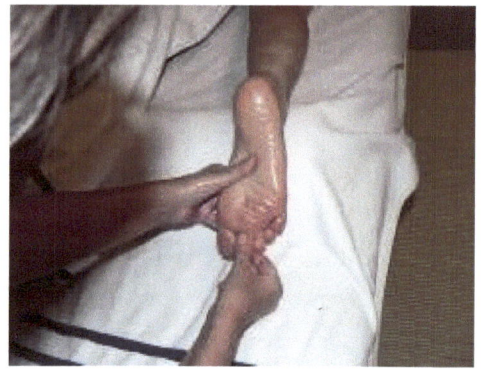

This practice involves the therapist applying pressure on the specific reflex zones on your feet in order to induce a healing response in corresponding areas of your body. This massage therapy was invented by Europeans in the late 1800s.

Reflex zones are essentially areas that are connected to other parts of your body. They're present on your hands, feet, and ears. The theory behind this massage therapy is that you can affect the nerves that carry signals to various parts of your body by applying pressure to reflex zones.

Some of the benefits of this type of massage therapy include improved circulation and relaxation.

Although many massage therapists have insight into reflexology, the best option is to find a reflexologist who is also a massage therapist in order to fully experience the benefits of this therapy.

Sports Massage

Sports massage is somewhat similar to deep tissue massage therapy, simply because it also focuses on reaching the deeper layers of your muscles.

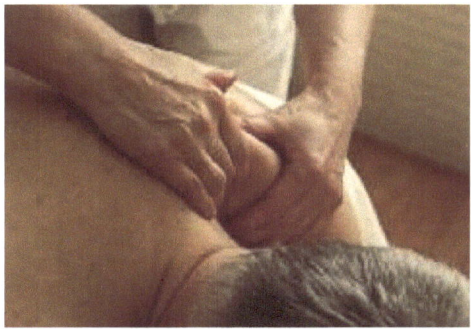

As the name suggests, this type of massage is geared towards any kind of athlete. It doesn't matter if you're a professional athlete or work out 3-4 days a week, as long as you're engaging in physical activity often, then you can benefit from this massage.

Massage therapists use different techniques during sports massage, and the therapist will focus on specific areas of your body that are stressed and overused from repetitive movements.

Not only will this type of massage put you in a state of relaxation and offer pain relief, but it can also be of benefit before a sports event, such as a marathon. If you're preparing for a specific event, then you need to add sports massage therapy into your preparation regimen, because it will improve you flexibility and endurance, reduce fatigue, and help prevent injuries.

Watsu

Watsu is also known as aquatic massage, and refers to an aquatic bodywork treatment usually done in a private heated pool.

Watsu was created by an aquatic bodyworker and poet named Harold Dull. This massage technique was discovered in the early 1980s, and was based on shiatsu therapy. This treatment is fairly unique and is something that you should definitely experience at least once. Watsu is known for helping you deal with chronic pain, stress related disorders, and postural imbalances.

It involves the therapist using a number of techniques to mobilize and stretch your soft tissues and joints. Because of the low gravity and warm water, a Watsu session will allow you to enter a state of deep relaxation.

Lymph Massage

Also referred to as lymphatic drainage, lymph massage was designed to help eliminate your body's waste. Lymphatic massage is typically the treatment of choice for swollen tissues as it helps remove proteins and waste products from the affected area and reduce the swelling.

Lymphedema

Lymphatic massage is technique that was developed in Germany, as a treatment for a condition known as lymphedema, which is described as an accumulation of fluids that sometimes occurs after lymph nodes are removed as part of a surgical procedure. It is also a condition that can develop at any time during an individual's life. The cause of this condition is currently unknown.

However, what is known is that lymphatic massage is proven to be quite effective when it comes to treating lymphedema.

It should be noted that this type of message is not medically recommended for people who are suffering from any condition other than lymphedema.

Relaxation

Lymphatic massage is especially relaxing and pleasant because it helps reduce pain all over the body. According to the International Alliance of Healthcare Educators, this particular massage therapy promotes general wellness, vitality, and healing.

Healing After Surgery

Lymph drainage massages is supportive of healing following surgery as regenerates tissues to reduce scarring that occurs as a result of surgical incisions. This therapy also reduces swelling, regenerates tissues and cells, and helps to detox the body, as reported by the International Alliance of Healthcare Educators.

Lymph massage should take place no sooner than six weeks following surgery and after a doctor has given approval.

Improved Breastfeeding

Breastfeeding complications as result of improper latching may include sore nipples, engorged breasts, and pain.

Lymphatic massage can help reduce the swelling that results from engorgement and help to ameliorate plugged ducts, resulting in less pain of the nipples and breasts, and leading to better breastfeeding.

Improved Immune System Functioning

The immune system is intricately tied to the lymphatic system, so much so that when the flow of lymphatic materials slows down, it actually weakens your immunity.

Lymph massage helps improve immune function and stimulates the production of antibodies that help fight off infection and disease and it goes further to reduce inflammation inside the body that is linked to various chronic conditions, such as arthritis.

A lymph massage is very gentle and not at all painful. A typical session lasts 45 to 60 minutes.

Healing Touch/Energy Healing

Healing touch is an energy therapy that revolves around the use of gentle hand techniques in order to help re-pattern the energy field of the patient, thus helping him or her accelerate healing of the mind, body, and spirit.

This massage therapy is based on a theory that people are fields of energy that constantly interact with other people and the environment. Healing touch therapy focuses on helping restore harmony to your energy system.

Amma

Amma is a form of massage therapy that is based on the principles of Chinese medicine that date back around 5,000 years.

Amma massage therapy is a mixture of deep tissue manipulation and the application of touch, friction, and pressure to specific points of your body.

This technique will help loosen your muscles, connective tissues, and joints, which will allow your body to function properly.

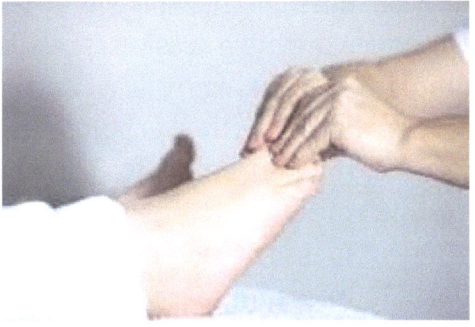

A great thing about Amma is that it's for everyone.

You don't have to be sick or suffering from ailments to take part in this massage therapy, you can book a session even if you're just feeling stressed out.

Amma therapy is used to treat and manage conditions like fractures, strains, sprains, as well as some chronic disorders.

Some of the most notable health benefits of Amma massage therapy include pain relief, fewer headaches, stress relief, reduced anxiety, and improved sleeping habits.

Balinese Massage

Balinese massage therapy was developed in Bali, and is based on the traditional medicine systems of China, India, and Southeast Asia.

Balinese massage is a full-body, deep-tissue treatment that is based on a mixture of gentle stretches, aromatherapy, reflexology, and acupressure. It is designed to stimulate the flow of blood in your body and help you achieve a state of deep relaxation.

Balinese massage therapists may use a number of different techniques during a session, such as pressure-point stimulation, stroking, rolling, and kneading, along with using essential oils to further promote the positive effects of the massage. If you're searching for a massage therapy that will help you relax, while offering you a chance to experience a variety of massage techniques, then you should definitely book a Balinese massage session.

Aqua Massage/Hydrotherapy

Aqua massage therapy doesn't involve the presence of a therapist. Instead, you have this massage in an aqua massage machine.

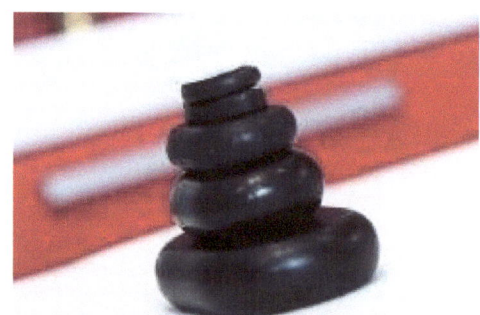

This machine looks very similar to a tanning bed. To prepare for an aqua massage, you only need to take off your shoes and lay down on the bed of the machine.

The cover of the machine, which consists of more than 36 water jets, will close over you and the massage will begin, as those jets stimulate all the muscles of your body.

Know that you won't get wet during an aqua massage, since there's a waterproof barrier between you and the cover of the machine. Most aqua massages last around 20 minutes to 1 hour.

Pregnancy Massage

Massage therapy can be of real benefit during pregnancy, as it can reduce anxiety, relieve muscle aches, and most importantly improve labor outcomes. Although the main goal of this massage is to improve your circulation and help you relax, it is also designed specifically to meet the needs of pregnant women.

Carrying a baby puts a lot of pressure on the shoulders, neck, back, and abdominal muscles. This can leave lasting effects on the posture, which is exactly why you should consider booking a prenatal massage session.

Benefits of Massage

Massage benefits the body, mind, and spirit in many ways.

General Health

- Promotes delivery of nutrients and oxygen cells within the muscle

- Helps remove waste products

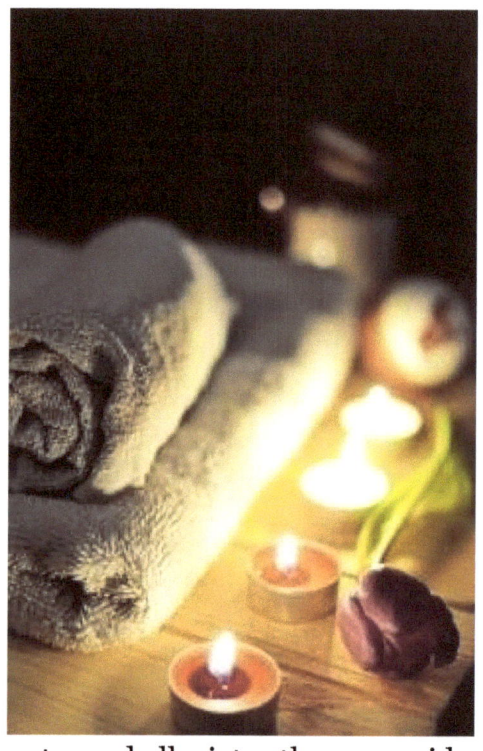

Circulatory effects help in treating inflammatory conditions, such as arthritis or edema through the use of lymphatic massage.

It also induces the relaxation response to lower heart rate, reduce blood pressure, respiration rate, and alleviates the many side effects of stress to promote a calm and healing environment within the body. Stress reduction and well-managed stress can also prevent the many chronic conditions associated with it, such as heart disease, depression, and anxiety.

Finally, it relaxes and calms the mind and spirit to make you more productive and generally better equipped to handle life.

Mobility And Movement

- Relaxes muscle tissue to decrease nerve compression, increase joint space, and improve range of motion leading to improved functioning and easier movement.

- Improved Athletic Performance & Recovery

It doesn't matter if you're a professional or amateur athlete, massage therapy can help improve your athletic performance.

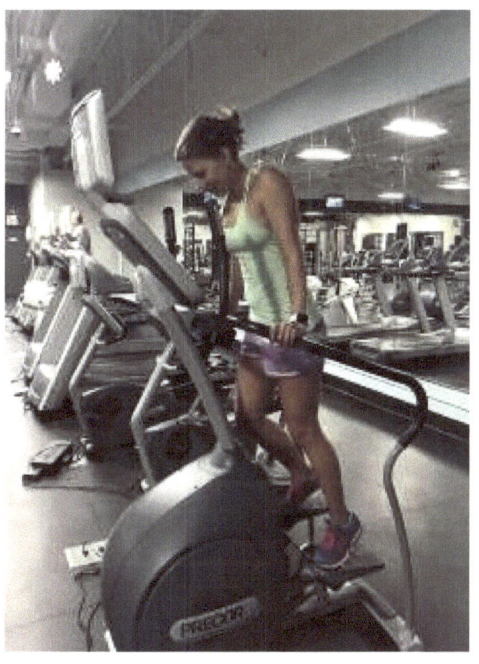

Deep tissue and sports massages are more suitable for athletes. Thanks to the fact that massage therapy has such a strong effect on your blood circulation, this practice will help reduce soreness, relieve muscle tension, help you recover faster and improve your overall performance in the gym or on the field.

Medical Conditions Helped By Massage

Enhanced Blood Flow And Blood Circulation

Improved circulation is one of the most notable health benefits of many types of massage techniques. Enhanced blood flow occurs as a result of regularly taking part in massage therapy.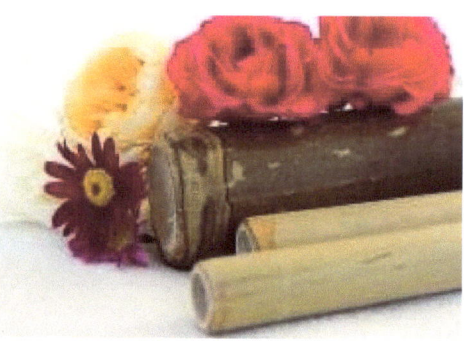
If you're suffering from poor circulation, then you may experience some discomforts like fatigue, cold feet and hands, pooling of fluid in your extremities, and accumulation of lactic acid in your muscles.

By improving your circulation, you will make sure that the bloodstream delivers oxygen to all parts of your body. This will have an incredibly positive effect on your overall health. It's also worth noting that by improving your blood circulation, you will lower your blood pressure levels.

Migraines and Headaches

Many people suffer from migraines and chronic headaches. Suffering from these conditions can be quite exhausting, since it often leads to lack of sleep and higher stress levels. This is exactly why many people turn to massage therapy in order to experience headache relief.

During most massage sessions, the therapist will partially focus on your head, shoulders, and neck, which will decrease the discomfort you experience as a result of headaches.

Additionally, when you get a massage, your therapist will work on relaxing relevant trigger points, which greatly reduces the chances of suffering from headaches or migraines.

Diabetes

Diabetes is a disease marked by damage to insulin production of the pancreas and features various symptoms, including excessive thirst, eye, heart, kidney and nerve damage, frequent urination, and thickening of fascia that surrounds organs and muscles.

Massage can help those with both type 1 and type 2 diabetes in numerous ways. First, it promotes relaxation, which improves all of the body's internal functions. Second, massage improves circulation, which helps promote more efficient uptake of insulin. Massage also improves mobility, joint motion, and decreases stiffness.

Parkinson's Disease

When an individual is suffering from Parkinson's disease, their central nervous system slowly begins to deteriorate. When your nerve cells die, your movement becomes affected. People who are suffering from Parkinson's disease often experience shaking and tremors, as well as uncoordinated movement.

There are some medications that can help reduce these symptoms, but it's better if you throw massage therapy into the mix. Massage therapy can help reduce muscle spasms, which are present in people with Parkinson's. It can also improve the state of your nervous system and help you get more quality sleep.

Heart Health

Excessive stress can cause numerous health problems, including cardiac arrhythmias. Additionally, high blood pressure will increase the risk of a heart attack.

Thankfully, massage therapy is known for both stabilizing your blood pressure and reducing stress. According to the American Massage Therapy Association, massage significantly decreases heart rate, systolic blood pressure, and diastolic blood pressure. These are the major reasons that getting massages regularly can significantly improve your heart health.

Healthy Blood Pressure

The scary thing about high blood pressure is that it has absolutely no symptoms, which is why it's often referred to as the silent killer. This is exactly why you need to make sure you check your blood pressure often, especially as you get older.

There are a few ways to stave off high blood pressure, such as exercising, eating healthy and getting massages regularly. Massage therapy is known for lowering blood pressure, which will in turn decrease your risk of suffering from a stroke, kidney failure, or a heart attack.

Fatigue

Every person experiences fatigue from time to time. Although fatigue isn't a cause for too much concern, as it usually goes away after you rest up, it can be a symptom of chronic fatigue syndrome, and it can certainly significantly lower your quality life.

Individuals who suffer from this syndrome can experience extreme fatigue for extended time periods, which can greatly affect their lifestyle. Massage therapy is currently one of the best alternative treatments for the symptoms of, fatigue and chronic fatigue syndrome.

PTSD

Soldiers aren't the only people who can suffer from Post Traumatic Stress Disorder. In fact, anyone who has ever experienced a severe trauma, such as abuse, crime or grief and loss can suffer from PTSD. The usual symptoms of this disorder include a feeling of detachment, chronic pain, anger, insomnia, severe anxiety, nightmares, and flashbacks.

You experience these symptoms due to imbalances in certain brain chemicals caused by stress that results from extreme trauma. Thankfully, engaging in massage therapy regularly is an efficient way to restore balance to these brain chemicals, and to help reduce PTSD symptoms.

Asthma And Bronchitis

Even if you're not suffering from asthma, you probably have a hard time taking a deep breath when faced with a stressful situation.

However, just imagine what it's like for the people suffering from asthma.

Considering that massage therapy is known for relaxing the respiratory muscles used in breathing, your life can change for the better if you start getting massages regularly. Aromatherapy massages are especially helpful for people suffering for asthma, with the help of certain essential oils that help improve respiration and promote healthier breathing.

Recovery From Surgery

Surgery to fix a specific health problem is very important, but so is the recovery process. Proper post-surgery rehabilitation is essential if you want to start feeling as you did when you were healthy.

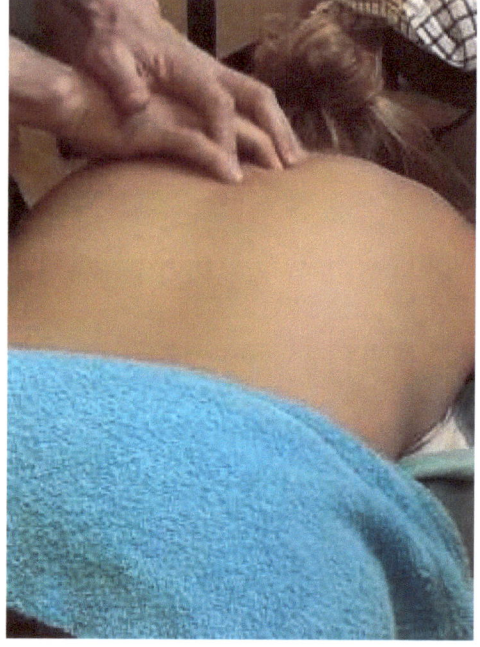

Massage therapy is an excellent way to make sure nutrients and blood reach the area of your body affected by the surgery and help in repairing the soft tissue.

Additionally, by getting massages, you will ensure that less scar tissue develops on your skin, such as the case with lymphatic massage. By improving circulation, the rehabilitating areas of your body will heal at a faster pace.

Cancer and Cancer Treatment

Oncology massage is a modified form of massage that's purpose is to safely address complications of cancer, side effects of cancer treatment and to support the patient in anyway needed.

An oncology massage therapists receive specialized training in understanding the disease itself and the many ways it can affect the body along with the side effects of various types of cancer treatment, such as chemotherapy, radiation, surgery, and medication.

A skilled therapist will modify massage techniques to meet the individual needs of the patient, in adaptation of their side effects and the various ways they are affected by the disease.

Insomnia

Due to chronic pain or high stress levels, it can be nearly impossible to get a good night's sleep. Watching the clock tick at night while you're wide-awake can be extremely frustrating. Starting off the day when you know that you haven't gotten enough sleep can also raise your stress levels, thus making your insomnia even more intense.

Insomnia is linked with increased risk of anxiety, depression, and memory loss. It is also one of the main causes of industrial disasters, medical errors, and car crashes.

Even though there are pills that will help you sleep, taking prescription medication can be addictive. Instead of taking sleeping pills to fix your insomnia problem, try getting regular massages.

Massages by a trained therapist can help alter the balance of neurochemicals in the brain, increasing expression of GABA (a key neurotransmitter for promoting restfulness) along with endorphins, which are key brain chemicals to combat the effect of adrenalin on the body, seeking to calm down neurons as the day progresses.

By informing your therapist about your insomnia issues, you will receive a massage tailored to help you deal with this condition. Massage therapy is a great way to become more relaxed, reduce your stress levels, and relieve pain. All of this will help make your insomnia go away.

One way to address insomnia more effectively is to hire a therapist that will come to your home close to your bedtime as possible, to really relax you and prepare the body for a good night's sleep.

Immunity Health

Having a strong immune system will help keep you safe from a number of different diseases. Most people have an incredibly weak immune system, mostly due to their lifestyle they lead. If you're always dealing with a lot of stress and not eating properly, then your immune system will gradually start losing its ability to protect your body from harmful microorganisms.

Massage therapy is known for increasing the presence of your body's natural white blood cells, which will help you fight against infection and bacteria.

Dr. Gail Ironson, of the University of Miami, completed a study with a group of HIV positive men being given a 45-minute massage, five days a week over the course of a month.

These men saw a serotonin increase and an increase in the white blood cells that are viewed as our immune system's first line of defense.

As it heightens the immune systems response, massage is a natural painkiller. Studies have shown that just one massage will have an immediate benefit on your immune system, while regular massages offer a cumulative long-term benefit.

Massage lowers stress hormone levels, while increasing white blood cell counts. It's a highly effective therapy for boosting immunity. It is one of the most enjoyable and affordable methods of staying healthy.

Mental and Emotional Health Benefits

The Touch Research Institute at the University of Miami has led many studies on the benefits of massage for mental health, and results show it to be beneficial for various conditions, including:

- Anorexia nervosa

- Depression

- Stress

- Anxiety

- And various other mental health conditions

Improved Mood

Anyone who has ever had a professional massage knows that there is a huge difference in how you feel before and after visiting a massage therapist. There are numerous reasons as to why massage is known for improving your mood, such as reduced stress and increased levels of feel good chemicals, including serotonin and endorphins. Not to mention that you will feel much happier when you reach a state of deep relaxation.

Anxiety

According to the American Massage Therapy Association, massage therapy is known for assisting in the reduction of anxiety symptoms.

Anxiety is basically caused by our body's natural response to danger, known as the fight or flight instinct.

However, this response to danger requires increased cortisol levels in order to make sure that your muscles are ready for the danger you're facing. Cortisol is also known as the 'stress hormone,' and high levels of it can lead to a number of health problems.

A massage therapist can target areas of your body where you carry anxiety symptoms, thus lowering your cortisol levels. Massage therapy will also improve your serotonin levels, which is a hormone that is known for elevating your mood.

According to the American Massage Therapy Association:

- Massage reduces trait anxiety and depression providing benefits similar to those in magnitude as psychotherapy

- Massage increases neurotransmitters that are associated with lowering anxiety and decrease hormones that play a key role in increasing anxiety

- Lowers anxiety in cancer patients

- Lowers anxiety and depression in military veterans

- Provides relaxation

According to the AMTA 2015 consumer survey, 33% of responders reported getting a massage for stress reduction and relaxation.

It's no secret that massage therapy can help you relax. In fact, that's one of the main reasons why most people even choose to get a massage. When the muscles in your body are 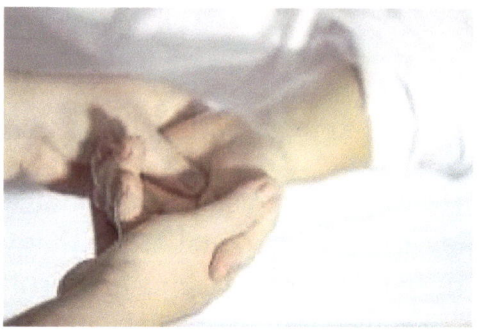 tense, you can experience digestive problems, sleeplessness, and headaches.

All massage therapy techniques were designed specifically to help relax your tense muscles, thus making you reach a state of deep relaxation. Achieving this state will provide you with improved emotional health, as well as better focus and memory.

Lower Stress Levels

The AMTA notes that massage is the most widely used type of complementary and alternative medicine in hospitals today for stress reduction, and general wellbeing.

Stress is not always a bad thing. For example, if you're feeling energetic before an important meeting, then you're dealing with the good kind of stress. However, if you're constantly 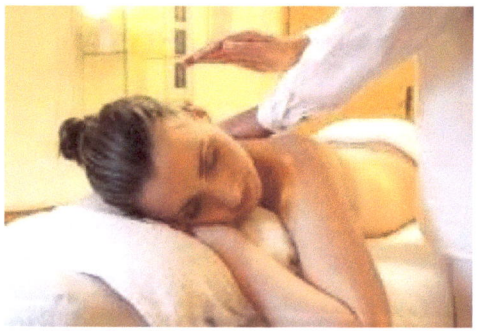 experiencing stress, and when it becomes a chronic state, then that's when you should start to worrying.

When you experience continuous or chronic stress, your body is constantly flooded with stress hormones and remains in a constant state of distress known as 'fight or flight', which can lead to numerous health problems, including higher blood pressure, insomnia, headaches, heart disease, chest pain, depression, anxiety, body aches and reduced quality of life. It's also worth mentioning that stress is known for worsening the symptoms of certain diseases.

By taking part in massage therapy, and especially on a regular basis, you will reduce your stress levels, which will in turn lower your risk of suffering from numerous health conditions. Massage also stimulates the productions of endorphins, also known as 'feel good' chemicals. Lowering your stress levels will not only improve your physical health, but it will also benefit your emotional health.

Researchers from the University of Miami School of medicine found that levels of the stress hormone cortisol were lowered by as much as 53% following just one session of massage.

According to Sandy Fritz, MS, NCMBT, author of a textbook line for therapeutic massage and director of the Health Enrichment Center in Lapeer, Michigan, "Research has shown that massage interfaces with the body's stress function," and "It helps to dampen the flight-or-fight response and activates dominance in the rest-and-restore system."

Depression

Massage therapy makes a great all natural addition to depression management. The American Massage Therapy Association acknowledges that massage therapy is able to reduce the symptoms of this condition.

The reason why massage therapy can reduce the risk of depression is that it lowers your cortisol levels by as much as 50%. Additionally, it raises levels of dopamine and serotonin, two neurotransmitters known for improving mood, and serotonin deficiency is a cause of major depression disorder.

As noted before, it also reduces depression in those who suffer from HIV.

Reduction In Anger And Aggression

You should never let stress lead you to your breaking point, as that can lead to depression, anxiety, anger, and aggression. However, you can avoid all of this simply by getting a massage once in a while. If you visit a massage therapist often, there probably won't be any chance for your stress levels to increase drastically.

Pain Conditions Helped By Massage

In a 2015 consumer survey, 91% of people surveyed agreed that massage was effective in reducing their pain.

Muscle Tension

Although some people experience muscle tension in the neck, back and shoulders from exercising too much, most experience it due to excessive sitting. Improper posture while standing and sitting is one of the main causes of chronic back pain.

Thankfully, massage therapy is able to help you by relaxing your tense muscles and improving your flexibility.

Chronic Back Pain

A 2011 study published in the ***Annals of Internal Medicine,*** evidence showed massage to be very effective for those who suffer from chronic back pain.

Chronic back pain is actually one of the most common reasons people get a massage, no matter its cause, be it poor posture, work related and other injuries, stress or carrying heavy items.

Fibromyalgia

Fibromyalgia is a very painful condition that affects the nerves of the body and makes life quite difficult for those suffering with it. Various massage therapies can help.

Trigger point therapy targets the most painful spots, which are located in bands of muscle fibers. This type of massage deactivates these areas by targeting trigger points identified to be the source of most pain, and uses pressure applied with the fingertip to massage them.

Swedish massage helps fibromyalgia patient alleviate stress. This in turn, helps promote relaxation, and general wellbeing that helps with pain management.

Myofascial release is a form of massage that applies gentle pressure to connective tissue, and helps to ease fibromyalgia pain and restore motion by elongating muscle fibers.

Hot-stone massage promotes relaxation and stress relief, thereby helping fibromyalgia sufferers improve their wellbeing, quality of life and reduce pain.

Passive stretching is a practice where external force is placed on a limb in order to move it into a new position. Those who suffer from fibromyalgia will have very stiff joints, which are caused by constant muscle spasms featured within this condition. Passive stretching helps to gentley move extremities in the same direction to loosen tight joints and muscles.

Sports massage can also benefit those with fibromyalgia as it releases stress and tension that builds up in the soft tissues of the body during physical activity. Sports massage also boosts blood circulation, reduces heart rate and blood pressure, increases lymph flow, improves flexibility, and eases pain.

If you have fibromyalgia, it's a good idea to find a massage therapist experienced in dealing with it. One example is the clinical massage therapist who works in a medical facility or hospital, as these are experts in various medical conditions, including fibromyalgia and how it affects the body, so they will be able to create a sound and effective treatment plan.

Arthritis & Rheumatoid Arthritis

Suffering from arthritis can limit your normal activities. Thankfully, massage therapy is known for reducing pain associated with this condition, as well as increase mobility for people suffering from arthritis.

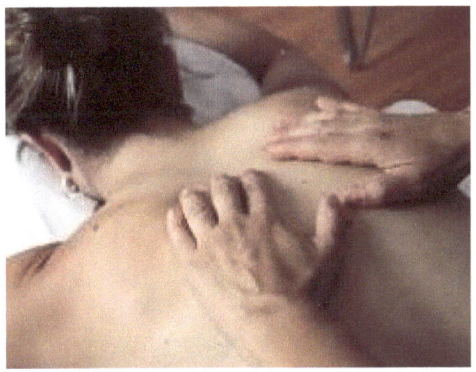

Regular massages could improve grip strength, relieve pain, and reduce anxiety in people suffering from this condition.

Various massage therapies can help with arthritis; you can discuss options that are most fitting for your condition with your therapist:

- Swedish

- Deep Tissue

- Hot Stone

- Ayurvedic

- Amma

- Thai Massage

- Lomi Lomi

- Myofascial Release

- Reflexology

- Rolfing

- Shiatsu

- Trigger Point

Frozen Shoulder

If you're having difficulty lifting your arms high, then you may be suffering from a frozen shoulder, or adhesive capsulitis. This condition is marked by soreness and stiffness within the shoulder joint, and is considered to be very painful and debilitating. Frozen shoulder affects 5% of the population.

Basically, having a frozen shoulder means that the connective tissue around your shoulder's tendons, ligaments, and bones became tighter.

Regular massage therapy and other bodywork modalities help treat this condition and alleviate the pain caused by it. Not only will it help with pain relief, but regular massages will also improve range of motion.

According to one study (Page, et al), deep friction massage can help frozen shoulder. Therapeutic massage techniques including trigger point therapy, stretching and joint mobilization and myofascial release either applied individually or in combination have shown positive results in alleviating frozen shoulder symptoms.

Massage techniques strive to release stiffness, boost blood and oxygen circulation, release locked-up muscles, and improve movement. A qualified massage therapist can create a treatment plan that consists of multiple sessions designed to unlock the stiff shoulder and restore the body's normal range of motion.

Sciatica

If you start experiencing pain from your lower back all the way down through your leg, then you may have damaged your sciatic nerve. This is one of the longer nerves found in the body, which is why the pain is so noticeable.

In sciatica, the tightening of the piriformis muscles in the back places undue stress on the nerve roots and massage helps to loosen those muscles, and also prevents irritation and pinching.

Furthermore, massage helps stimulate the release of the body's natural painkillers, known as endorphins to provide relief for sciatica symptoms, including throbbing pain in the foot and burning sensations in the legs.

Jeff Smoot, vice president of the American Massage Therapy Association says that trigger point therapy is the best type of massage for sciatica.

Trigger point therapy applies pressure to the irritated and inflamed areas in the piriformis muscle, glutes, and lower back. Typically, progress can be seen by the 4th session, with treatments being given 7 to 10 days apart.

Rotator Cuff Syndrome

Your rotator cuff is extremely important to the body because it offers extraordinary range of motion in the shoulder. The rotator cuff is a group of tendons and muscles that sits in the shoulders and 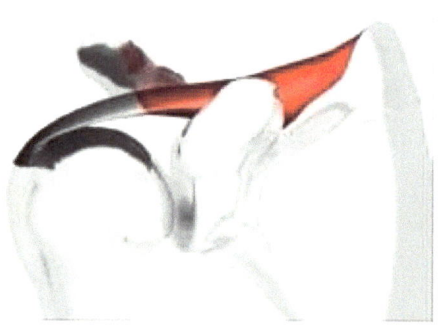 connects the upper arm to the shoulder blade.

If your rotator cuff is injured, you'll notice almost instantly. For example, you won't be able to throw a ball overhead or pick up something off a shelf. Because your rotator cuff muscles are surrounded by bones, the interior pressure of your shoulder socket will increase if your rotator cuff becomes injured.

This will cause the muscle tissue to start to fray, since it will stop receiving a lot of blood. By getting a massage, you'll increase blood flow to your rotator cuff muscles, thus helping them heal.

Muscle Sprains And Strains

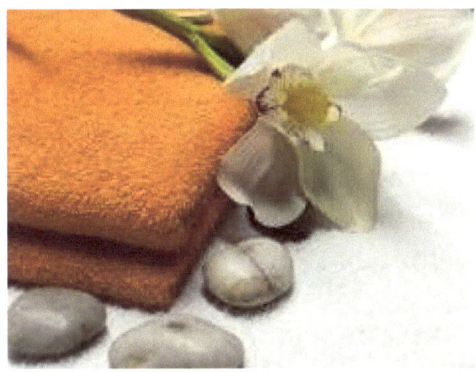

Massage therapy is a great way to efficiently treat muscle sprains and strains. This comes as no surprise considering that the massage therapist will spend all of their time during a session working on your soft tissues. Following a strain or a sprain, you will have to avoid engaging physical activity for several weeks, but thanks to massage therapy, you will fully recover after those weeks.

Myofascial Pain Syndrome

Myofascial pain syndrome is quite different from the muscle soreness you may feel after a challenging workout. One of the best ways to relieve myofascial pain is to get either a deep tissue or a hot stone massage.

It's worth noting that this syndrome is known to raise the risk of insomnia, depression, and anxiety. Thankfully, getting a massage suitable for relieving the symptoms of myofascial pain syndrome will help reduce these symptoms as well.

Effective Types Of Massage For Myofascial Syndrome

Deep tissue massage targets knots and helps to release chronic tension by using stroking techniques against the grains of the muscles.

Placing deep pressure on the fascia, the protective layer that surrounds bones, muscles and joints, deep tissue massage may feel uncomfortable during the session, but provides lasting long-term benefits for the condition.

Hot stone massage helps reach deeper layers of the muscles to reduce myofascial pain while at the same time increasing relaxation and reducing stress. The warm stones work to improve blood circulation, and offer a sedative effect that helps relieve chronic pain.

Cancer

Massage therapy not only helps with pain related to cancer, and treatments, but it also helps fight the stress and anxiety associated with cancer diagnosis. On top of that, it will also help to manage treatment side effects such as fatigue and nausea.

HIV

Massage therapy can help people suffering from HIV primarily by strengthening their immune system, thus helping them fight the disease. Additionally, it can help relieve certain HIV/AIDS symptoms, such as inflammation, body tension, cramps, and muscle spasms.

Sports Injuries

If a damaged muscle is massaged right away, there is a high chance of an extremely fast recovery. If you're an athlete and have suffered an injury, but want to get back to working out quickly, then you should make sure to visit a massage therapist or a physical therapist as soon as possible. Massages are a great way to recover from sports injuries.

Carpal Tunnel Syndrome

If you experience numbness, tingling, or pain in your hands and wrists then you might be suffering from carpal tunnel syndrome. This syndrome usually affects the individual's dominant hand, which can negatively affect your movement.

Getting a massage tailored for fixing your problems will carpal tunnel syndrome will greatly reduce the symptoms associated with this condition.

Massage As a Low-Risk Treatment

Massage has no side effects; it is a noninvasive low risk treatment option for many conditions and general wellness.

Massage is also an excellent preventative measure, as an excellent tool in support of stress as it ensures that chronic stress does not cause the many chronic conditions it is associated with and supports your overall wellness, and therefore quality of life.

Does Massage Hurt?

Normally, massage should not hurt, though this can depend on the condition being treated, with some discomfort being normal and a part of enjoying long-term relief and benefits.

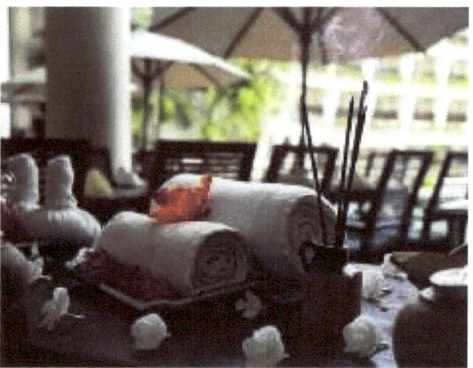

Some people may experience some discomfort following their first or second session, but overall the purpose of massage is for it to feel good during and make you better after a session.

If the typical relaxation massage hurts, it is important to tell the therapist performing it immediately, it is likely just a matter of applying less pressure.

Remember that the massage is for you, and should be a pleasurable experience.

Conditions Where Massage Is Not Advised

Most people can benefit from massage, but it is not appropriate if you have:

- Burns

- Healing wounds

- Taking blood-thinning medication or have a bleeding disorder

- Deep vein thrombosis

- Fractures

- Severe osteoporosis

- Severe thrombocytopenia

Always advise your massage therapist, and they are always supposed to ask you, of any medical conditions you have.

Tips For Finding A Good Massage Therapist

Finding a good massage therapist is really important if you want to truly experience all the health benefits that you can gain from massage therapy. If you've never gotten a massage before, know that you won't be able to recognize a good therapist from a bad one simply by judging how your session went.

First and foremost, they should be licensed and certified in the state where they practice.

Massage is not just random kneading of the 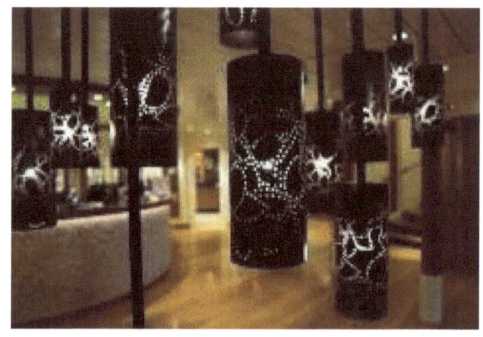 body, but requires education and a comprehensive understanding of the human body, anatomy, and pressure points.

Knowledgeable and experienced massage therapists know exactly what to do, and where and how to apply pressure to yield the best results.

Expert massage therapists also understand the connection between certain conditions and massage, for example, if you are pregnant the massage therapist will use specific techniques to ensure your health and safety, as not all massage forms are appropriate for pregnant women. Well-trained therapists also understand how massage affects various medical conditions, and injuries.

To make sure you're getting the real deal, you should check if the massage therapist you're about to book a session with is certified, licensed and if available, reviews of their performance – both good and bad.

Reputable massage therapists are found in spas, health and fitness centers, massage clinics, hospitals, physical therapy centers, clinics, massage schools, and even online for in-home service.

Final Thoughts

Massage therapy is used to manipulate your soft body tissues with the goal of improving your overall health. There are many different massage techniques, such as Swedish massage, 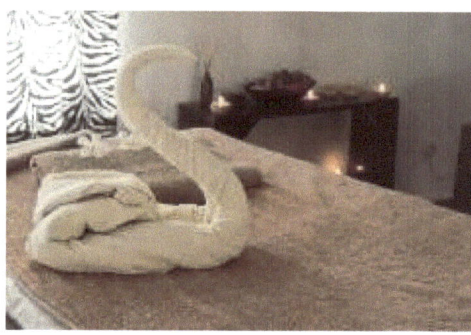 shiatsu, deep tissue massage, Watsu, hot stone massage, reflexology, Thai massage, Amma, aromatherapy massage, sports massage, and more.

All of these different techniques offer varying health benefits.

Some of the most notable general health benefits of massages include relaxation, improved blood circulation, lower blood pressure, pain relief, depression management, enhanced mood, improved heart health, lower stress levels, anger management, better sleep, and a general boost in overall wellness of mind, body and spirit.

Massage also helps in managing various chronic and acute medical ailments, along with pain conditions to speed up recovery and improve wellbeing.

With all of the health benefits it provides, massage therapy is considered to be one of the best forms of alternative medicine. It really can improve your quality of life, general health, and general wellness.

Other Relevant Books by This Author

If you would like to read more relevant books about this topic, here is a list of the CreateSpace links, titles and descriptions from this author:

https://www.createspace.com/5714434

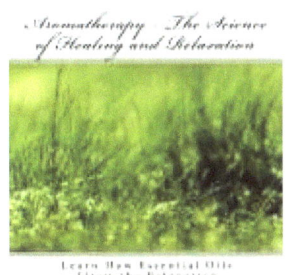

Aromatherapy - The Science of Healing and Relaxation

In my book *Aromatherapy – The Science of Healing and Relaxation*, we reveal the natural holistic methods issues and to relive stress through relaxation.

In particular we talk about:
• Aromatherapy - what it is and how it works
• Essential Oils – how the effects of certain aromas differs from others
• Recipes – how to make your own essential oil combinations

Aromatherapy

The results of The American Psychological Association's 2010 Stress in America survey showed that nearly 75% of Americans who responded to the survey believe their stress levels to be so high that they feel unhealthy.

Stress and anxiety reflect the reaction of the body and the mind when over stimulated.

Stress tends to reflect the physical responses of the body when coping with daily pressures, physical labor, a high-paced work environment, toxic relationships, and financial and emotional responsibilities, which exceed a person's ability to cope or manage. However, your sense of smell can help relieve stress by smelling certain aromas.

Essential Oils

When selecting oils to combat anxiety and stress, choose oils with relaxing, calming, and uplifting properties. The oils should soothe while shifting the awareness in a way that grounds and replenishes the constitution of the person being treated. The scents that work best for anxiety and stress relief tend to have light and bright floral, citrus, or woodsy scents.

The essential oils recommended for relaxation and mood adjustment may be blended with those recommended for managing stress and anxiety. Many of them are complementary scents with complementary therapeutic qualities.

Recipes

There are many ways to enjoy the benefits of essential oils. When selecting a method of application, the issue being treated must be considered along with the desired results.

For example:

==> Creams, ointments, and gels work best for treating injuries like bruises and cuts.

==> A massage oil works well for treating muscle aches and pains.

==> If the primary purpose of the treatment is to shift a person's mood in some way, incense or a diffuser may be the best option.

While you can buy certain combinations of oils, we include in our book several recipes and show you how you can make a unique essential oil tailored just to you.

Aromatherapy – The Science of Healing and Relaxation is a must-have book for those that are overstressed and starting to exhibit the effects of stress either through the development of physical or mental responses, or both. What you smell can make you feel better!

https://www.createspace.com/6414998

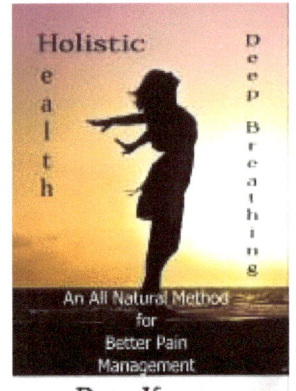

Deep Breathing to Help Relieve Chronic Pain: An All-Natural Method for Better Pain Management

Chronic pain is pain that lasts longer than six months and can't be cured, but can be treated and managed. The pain can range from mild to excruciating and can be either episodic or continuous.

According to WebMD, approximately 100 million Americans alone suffer from chronic pain; imagine the numbers worldwide!

Chronic pain can affect anyone at any age, for example, if you have a sports injury at a young age, the pain can sometimes follow you throughout life or you are 60 and diagnosed with arthritis … the stage I'm now at in my life having been diagnosed with osteoarthritis five years ago.

Often early injuries, present injuries, or other reasons end up causing chronic pain. Some people have certain genetic codes predispose them towards having chronic pain.

There are several conditions that cause chronic pain such as fibromyalgia, arthritis, neuropathy, carpal tunnel syndrome, migraines, and others.
You can also have an injury when you are younger and have chronic pain stemming from it but starting later on in life.

Chronic pain can be a result of repetition in body movement from a job and sometimes, people simply suffer from chronic pain syndrome whose cause cannot be identified. Regardless, it can have a mind of its own, flaring up for no apparent reason with science still not fully understanding why.

So the best treatment is to try and manage it. While many try medications, sometimes their side effects are worse that the pain they are trying to manage. Others go for a more holistic method of treatment like deep breathing. It is cheaper, can be done anytime, doesn't have harmful side effects, and in some cases can be just as effective.

In this book we explore how deep breathing can reduce the effects of chronic pain along with the other health benefits of deep breathing.

https://www.createspace.com/6837889

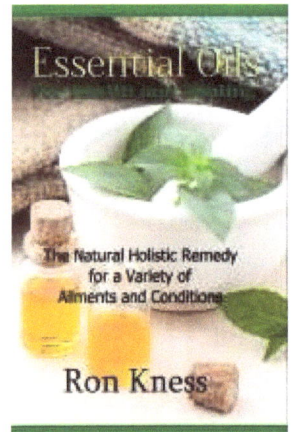

Essential Oils for Health and Healing: The Natural Holistic Remedy for a Variety of Ailments and Conditions

The use of essential oils for therapeutic purposes dates back to 6,000 years ago. The ancient Romans, Indians, Chinese, Greeks, and Egyptians all used them for hygienic, therapeutic, ritualistic, and spiritual purposes.

More than 2,500 years ago, Hippocrates noted that aromatic baths had a significant impact on the overall well-being of an individual.

During the early 19th century, essential oils started being present in western medicine practices, while later on in the century, both German and French medical professors started using them to fight infected wounds.

Some of the most popular uses of essential oils are inhalation, massaging essential oils into the skin, and mixing them with face creams and body lotions.

By applying essential oils properly, you'll experience a great alternative treatment for stress, fatigue, insomnia and many other health problems. When essential oils are used in a diffuser as aromatherapy, they are well known for improving mood and providing wonderful healing scents that promote general wellness and wellbeing.

Essential oils can not only help you with the health issues noted above, but could end up being your natural holistic remedy for:
- Headaches and migraines
- Joint aches and pains
- Chronic pain
- Menstrual irregularities
- Cuts, scrapes and burns
- Signs of aging and wrinkles
- Anxiety and depression

If you have never used essential oils before, get a starter kit and start using them. I think you'll be pleasantly surprised at just how beneficial they can be as a natural holistic cure.

About the Author

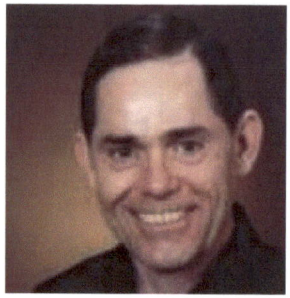

I have published over 125 books on Amazon for Kindle, CreateSpace and other publishing platforms.

While most of my books are on health and fitness in general, as I age (now 65) at the time of this writing) my topics of interest are geared toward aging baby boomers and older.

Besides my own writing, I also ghostwrite ebooks, books, reports, articles, blogs and do Kindle conversions for clients on a variety of topics.

Today my wife and I are retired from our careers and live in Gold Canyon, AZ. I now write as a retirement business where you'll find me happily sitting in my office typing away on my laptop as I work on my next book or ghostwriting project . . . that is if we are not traveling on a cruise ship - our new-found mode of travel.